VOLUMETRICS DIET

A Review of the Diet and Beginner's Step-by-Step Overview

Bruce Ackerberg

mindplusfood

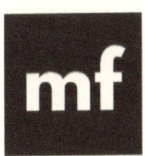

DISCLAIMER

By reading this disclaimer, you are accepting the terms of the disclaimer in full. If you disagree with this disclaimer, please do not read the guide.

All of the content within this guide is provided for informational and educational purposes only, and should not be accepted as independent medical or other professional advice. The author is not a doctor, physician, nurse, mental health provider, or registered nutritionist/dietician. Therefore, using and reading this guide does not establish any form of a physician-patient relationship.

Always consult with a physician or another qualified health provider with any issues or questions you might have regarding any sort of medical condition. Do not ever disregard any qualified professional medical advice or delay seeking that advice because of anything you have read in this guide. The information in this guide is not intended to be any sort of medical advice and should not be used in lieu of any medical advice by a licensed and qualified medical professional.

The information in this guide has been compiled from a variety of known sources. However, the author cannot attest to or guarantee the accuracy of each source and thus should not be held liable for any errors or omissions.

You acknowledge that the publisher of this guide will not be held

CONTENTS

INTRODUCTION

There is this prevailing notion that losing weight is expensive, time-consuming, and demands a lot of thought and effort. This is even backed by the fact that many who lose weight did so using highly rigid diet regimes.

But what if you were told that there is an easier way to shed extra weight?

Volumetrics Diet is an award-winning diet plan that is backed up by scientific studies regarding energy density. It has been ranked as the 6th out of the 32 participants in the Best Diets Overall category of the US News and World Report's Best Diet 2014.

It also ranked number 4 in the Best Diets for Healthy Eating category, number 5 in the Best Weight-loss Diets category, and number 8 in the Best Diabetes Diets category. Studies done by the creator of the Volumetrics diet, Barbara Rolls, also proved the effectiveness of this diet plan. Some of those studies have been published in the American Journal of Clinical Nutrition.

The Volumetrics diet plan is a proven and tested plan that mainly focuses on the energy density of foods taken in. It is more of an eating plan than a diet plan because participants are not prohibited to eat any type of food, but are actually recommended to eat more.

The rationale behind this is that a participant can eat more of very low-density foods, but must eat limited amounts of high-density foods. It primarily focuses on the idea of fullness, which means that foods with higher water and fiber content are recommended. Many nutritionists suggest this eating plan because it does not focus on deprivation and because of the fact that this diet plan changes the perception of individuals when it comes to food.

This book is written to help beginners understand the important details of Volumetrics. It includes a detailed definition of Volumetrics together with research conclusions that prove the effectiveness of this diet plan. The four food categories introduced by Barbara Rolls are also included to help the reader understand the concept of energy density in foods. It also contains a step-by-step process on how to start a Volumetrics diet.

A simple meal plan is given to give the reader an idea of what foods are usually taken in by a participant. It also gives a brief discussion of the importance of other nutrients such as protein. Aside from that, the 5th chapter of the book includes a detailed discussion of the food list. The list ranges from very low-density foods to high-density foods. Examples of each food category are also given.

An entire chapter will be devoted to recipes that you can prepare for Breakfast, Lunch, and Dinner. Nutrition facts of each recipe are also provided to help the reader calculate and keep track of their calorie consumption since that is the most consuming activity in this eating plan.

Thanks again for downloading this book. I hope you enjoy it!

PHASE 1: THE BASICS OF THE VOLUMETRICS DIET

B efore anything else, you have to be aware of what are signing up for. This diet only works if you have an understanding of its basic concepts and processes. As such, here are a few things about the diet that you need to know about.

What is the Volumetrics Diet?

Volumetrics is a diet plan that helps individuals choose healthy foods that they can eat and will satisfy them without gaining weight. It promotes satiety, the idea of "feeling full". It pays attention to the energy density of the foods which means that it relies on foods with lots of water content such as fruits and vegetables because they satisfy you without adding too many calories.

The trick in this diet is to eat the proper type and amount of foods that contain the right amount of calories, fat, protein, and carbohydrates that make people feel full. This diet plan boils down to the basics: low calories, low fat, and lots of fruits and vegetables.

Volumetrics eating plan is not a fast weight-loss diet program. Instead, it is a long-term eating plan that helps a participant develop a healthy lifestyle. The goal of this plan is to lose 5 to 10% of your weight in two weeks. That aim is more reasonable and sustainable than losing 10 pounds in a week.

This diet plan was a product of decades of research by a veteran Nutrition professor named Barbara Rolls, PhD. She spent 20 years studying the science of satiety and has written over 200 research articles. She also directs the laboratory for the study of Human Ingestive Behavior at the Pennsylvania State University. She has also studied eating behaviors and dietary patterns. She wrote the book "The Volumetrics Weight-Control Plan".

The volumetrics diet is one of the most popular and effective diet plans available. Its effectiveness is backed by studies done by different researchers. A study done by the Centers for Disease Control and Prevention showed that diets rich in low-energy-dense foods promote fullness and because they only contain a few calories, they promote weight loss. Another study done by the American Journal of Clinical Nutrition in 2002 shows that people who eat fruits and vegetables tend to lose more weight. It shows that a low-energy-dense diet is an effective way to drop pounds and keep them off.

Another study done in 2008 between two groups concluded that the group who ate high-density foods increased their body mass index more than that of the group who ate low-density foods. Studies suggest that decreasing energy density is a way to prevent weight gain and obesity in the short and long term.

Aside from the studies that back its effectiveness, the Volumetrics diet is ranked 6th in the Best Diets Overall 2014 category. It outperformed its competitors in being safe and healthy.

This diet plan is more of an approach to eating than a structured diet. It is a flexible plan that helps you recognize when you're full and gives you a chance to make smart choices about the foods you eat. Stress or emotional eating is also addressed in this diet plan. Here are some of the limits you have to follow regarding your food intake:

Calories must be minimized by 500 to 1000 calories from your usual daily intake.

Total fat must be limited to 20-30% of total calories.

Carbohydrates must comprise 55% or more of the total calories.

Fiber intake must amount to 20 to 30 grams per day.

The intake of added sugars, alcohol, and caffeine must be moderated.

Protein must be 15% of daily calories.

Adequate daily water intake is important. Women must drink up to 9 cups while men must drink up to 12 cups.

Salient Features
The Volumetrics Diet is unlike other weight-loss programs. As such, before you even consider implementing this kind of diet in your life, you need to know what sets it apart from the others, both good and bad.

Advantages
Build your own meal plan
Since there are no severe restrictions on what you can or can't eat, you can effectively follow the Volumetrics diet without being limited to a few food groups. Sure, there are some recommended food groups that you should consume and there are certain recipes that you may include in your daily meals (more on these later on).

However, this does not detract from the fact that you are in complete control over what you eat. On a more practical scale, this allows you to make better decisions on what you put on your body while also learning how to prepare food better.

By not removing personal agency from the meals, the Volumetrics diet works less like a chore and more like a lifestyle. After all, things are more achievable if you don't feel forced down a certain path.

So whether you like your meat, your pasta, or your desserts, you won't have to say goodbye to them.

It's a lifestyle—not a fad

A quick glance at a standard Volumetrics Diet will show you that it merely does away with fattening food, not depriving your body of the required quantity it needs to function normally every day.

Instead of cholesterol and sugars, your diet would comprise food rich in vitamins, minerals, and important nutrients such as body-building proteins.

This should allow you to manage your weight or even lose some while still getting the nutrients you need to go through a long, arduous day.

Sustainable

The biggest draw with this kind of diet plan is that it does not demand that you deprive yourself of yummy food. One of the biggest challenges in any diet is the constant struggle your mind has to deal with in order not to focus too much on hunger.

This can be mentally taxing which is why a lot of people abandon their diets altogether to satiate their hunger. The Volumetrics diet, on the other hand, only asks that you make changes as to the portions and proportions—you still get to enjoy food.

Nonetheless, this diet plan requires commitment. You'll need to keep your motivation and just keep pushing forward until the changes become so ingrained in you that they will require very little effort.

However, despite how good all of these sound, the Volumetrics diet does have some downsides. This is unavoidable as diet plans are designed to be done in a certain way, no matter how flexible they are.

Disadvantages
<u>You'll have to prepare your own food</u>
The effort to make sure that you eat healthy will be quite considerable with the volumetrics diet plan. Not only must you learn how to properly prepare food, but you must also learn how to count calories to make sure that you don't go beyond your body's daily caloric intake limit.

The long prep time for food and the tedium of keeping records and counting calories can be off-putting for people, especially those who are not detail-oriented.

<u>No rapid weight loss results</u>
If you're looking to lose a lot of weight overnight, this program is not for you.

It is guaranteed to work but it works slowly. This slow burn can give off the impression that the diet is not working which can be frustrating. However, considerable weight loss is possible if you can commit to the plan on a long-term basis.

PHASE 2: THE VOLUMETRICS FOOD LIST

The Volumetrics diet plan is divided into four categories. The first category is composed of very low-density foods, the second category is composed of low-density foods, the third category is made up of medium-density foods, and the fourth category is composed of high-density foods.

Very low density also called "free or anytime" foods are those with low energy density because of their high-water content.
Some examples of these are fruits like raspberries, peaches, apples, and the like, broth-based soups, and non-starchy vegetables.

Low-density foods are great sources of energy and fiber. These foods contain complex carbohydrates that are important in our body.

Low-density foods include lean proteins, low-fat dairy, tofu, vegetarian chili, shrimp, olives, whole grains, cereals, and pasta.
Medium energy density foods contain low amounts of fiber but a decent amount of fat. Intake of medium-density foods must be limited because of their high cholesterol, but low essential vitamins contents.

Examples of medium-density foods are bread, cheese, fat-free baked snacks, frozen yogurt, turkey breast, Italian dressing, bagel, hard pretzels, raisins, angel food cake, pork, and beef.

High-density foods have high fat and low water and fiber contents, which make them unsuitable for dieters.

They also contain food preservatives and added sugar which is strictly prohibited. Nutritionists suggest that the consumption of this food category must be minimized.

Foods included in this category are chocolates, cookies, butter, candies, oils, nuts, baked potato chips, tortilla chips, croissants, and bacon.

PHASE 3: EMBRACING THE LIFESTYLE

Aside from being a diet plan, Volumetrics also aims to change our eating habits.

Before starting any diet plan, one must first understand the basics about it to avoid any problems. Keep in mind that this diet plan focuses more on calorie density or the amount of calories a certain food contains. Familiarizing yourself with the terms and ideas of this diet plan will guide you in achieving your goals.
Steps to finding success with the Volumetrics diet

To be able to maintain a healthy lifestyle with this diet plan, here are the steps on how to get through it and achieve success:

Learn Volumetrics Recipes

After understanding the calorie intake, you can now start searching for recipes that will suit your taste. The good thing about this diet plan is that no type of food is prohibited; what you only need to do is to limit your intake. This means that you have plenty of recipe choices though it is recommended to eat more fruits and vegetables. There's an entire chapter for recipes included in the later parts of the book.

Read the Volumetrics Food List.

There are so many different kinds of food and food items out there so it's best to develop your own food list depending on your taste and calorie needs (which also depend on your level of activity and target weight loss goals). You'll be using this food list when preparing your shopping list and your meal plans.

Reading the food list can help you identify portions of food with specific caloric contents. The key to being successful in this diet plan is knowing how to properly measure food portions. The food list usually starts with foods that have very low-calorie contents to foods with high-calorie density.

You'll learn more about this in the next chapter.

Prepare meal plans.
After learning all you need to know about this diet plan, you can now start creating a meal plan. Start by choosing or creating healthy recipes and then make your shopping list. Make sure to include lots of vegetables and fruits. Your food list must contain more low-density foods.

In planning your meals, you have to compute your individual calorie needs. Knowing that will help you in planning your meals since you have to divide your calorie requirements into 5 meals. Calorie requirements must be divided into the following meals: breakfast, lunch, dinner, and snacks.

Understand energy density.
Since the focus of this diet plan is the intake of calories, learning the food categories enumerated in the second chapter would be helpful. Volumetrics diet plan requires you to take 1,600 calories per day, so you must estimate your calorie needs based on your height and activity level. To be able to lose 1 pound per week, you have to reduce your calorie intake by 500.

Stay on track when eating out.
When you're eating in a restaurant, you have to focus on controlling the portion of the food you eat. It is best to start with a soup or salad so that you can properly control eating the main

dish. Always remember, to eat larger portions of foods with lower density and smaller portions of foods with high density.

Maintenance.

Volumetrics diet plan is a long-term plan so you will need to be patient before you see the results. To maintain such results, you have to learn how to listen to hunger signals. Eat when you are hungry but always make sure not to overindulge on any food. Keeping a record of the foods you ate and the physical activities you did is also recommended.

This is to keep track of your meal plan and to make necessary improvements. Hitting the gym is not required, but basic exercises such as walking are highly recommended. Walking for 30 minutes a day is sufficient exercise to partner with your Volumetrics eating plan.

What to Expect with the Volumetrics Diet

Gradual Weight Loss

Unlike other diet plans, the Volumetrics Diet system does not promise massive weight loss within a short period of time. It is focused more on changing the quality of the food being consumed by the body. This should allow the body to burn through its stored nutrients efficiently.

This means that your body should gradually shed off its extra fat and replace that mass with leaner, tougher muscles. Combined with a workout, the amount of weight you lose will increase and the physique you gain will be achieved in a shorter period of time.

Improved Health

By replacing every harmful substance in your diet with healthier alternatives, you give your body the opportunity it needs to improve itself. By lowering the saturated fat content in the body, the Volumetrics diet can also help in lowering your blood pressure as well as increasing your insulin levels.

This means that the chances of your body developing life-threatening conditions like Type 2 Diabetes and heart disease are drastically lowered. Also, improving your body's resistance means that you are less likely to be bogged down by simpler conditions like the flu.

<u>Healthy Habits</u>
Aside from the physical benefits, the Volumetrics Diet plan has the mental effect of allowing you to slowly embrace a healthier lifestyle. The plan is meant to be implemented on a long-term basis to ensure the best possible results. At best, you can expect to follow your own Volumetrics diet plan over a period spanning an entire year at least.

This will provide enough time for you to pick up several health-conscious habits. From checking on the nutritional content of your food to even properly cooking and storing them, habits like these are what make any kind of lifestyle healthier. In time, you will be able to make healthy decisions purely on instinct.

Frequently Asked Questions
So, what else should you know about the Volumetrics Diet plan? Here are some of the more frequently asked questions (FAQs) regarding this weight loss plan.

Is it expensive?
The volumetrics diet is only as expensive as you want it to be. In fact, this is one of the diet plans that will go easy on your weekly grocery budget. The goal is just to replace your less-healthy food items with healthier ones. You just might be surprised at how cheaper certain fruits and vegetables are compared to meat and dairy products.

Is it difficult to follow?
No. The volumetrics diet plan requires that you only master how to properly prepare your food as well as control the portions of your meal. You do not need to exercise in order to make this plan effective. However, constant physical activity does amplify the results of the diet.

Also, there is no need for constant meetings with dietitians and nutritionists with this diet. You can do this all on your own. What is just required for you is to be as disciplined as possible in following the plan.

How Flexible is the Volumetrics Plan?
This diet plan can work with any existing health condition. If you are already adopting a Vegan diet, you are practically adopting 50% of the diet already.

Also, this diet is helpful for people suffering from a number of medical conditions such as heart disease, sleep apnea, arthritis, and diabetes. In some cases, this diet might even reduce your dependence on certain medications.

That being said, however, it is best to consult with a doctor first before implementing this plan. They would know if this diet is compatible with your medications and will provide you with the necessary nutrition.

What happens if you fail to follow the Volumetrics Diet Plan?
Humans, after all, are not known for their infallibility. There will be times when you will overeat especially if you are invited for dinner at a restaurant.

The first thing to do is to stop feeling sorry for yourself. You have to understand that it is easy to go beyond the daily caloric intake, especially during special occasions. The last thing you want to do is to beat yourself for food you have already eaten.

Next, you have to backtrack and remember what kind of food you ate the previous day. Most likely, people overeat during lunch and dinner as the body is at its hungriest in these instances.

Perhaps it was 3 extra slices of pizza this time. Or maybe it was that bowl of Popcorn you ate while binge-watching Netflix. Either way, you have to recall what you ate and pinpoint exactly where you overate to prevent similar occurrences.

Lastly, you have to adjust either your intake for that day or the amount of work you have to exert. Both strategies work in helping your body burn through that extra fat while also not adding more to it.

PHASE 4: MAKING YOUR OWN FOOD LIST

Your food list must be composed of more low-density foods such as lentil soups and oatmeal pancakes. The inclusion of high density and medium-density foods must be limited. Your food list must contain the following:

Fruits and vegetables
This is the most important food that you must include in your list. Fruits and vegetables are full of water and fiber. Choosing vegetables and fruits that have high water content such as tomatoes, broccoli, watermelons, and strawberries is a must because water makes the food bulkier, which allows you to stay fuller for a longer time. Adding vegetables to other dishes that do not normally require such vegetables is a good way to recreate a recipe. Aside from that, adding a salad dish to a meal reduces the calories consumed.

Lean meats
Lean meats are also important in a balanced meal plan. Lean meat is a great source of protein, essential vitamins, and minerals. In choosing meats, pork must be minimized, if not avoided. The visible fats in the meat must also be trimmed. Aside from that, poultry and fishes must be given more importance because of their low-calorie content.

Whole grains

Whole grains are the usual foods for breakfast because of their high fiber contents. It is recommended to choose whole wheat over refined all-purpose flour. Researchers also suggest that making your own food is better than consuming pre-packaged ones because sometimes preservatives are already added to the latter. Whole grains include pasta, brown rice, breads, and cereals.

Dairy

Low-fat dairy is a great source of calcium, which is essential in improving the health of your bones. Examples of low-fat dairy are milk, yogurt, and cheese. Take them in moderation. In choosing dairy products, one must choose non-fat or fat-free products because they contain fewer calories.

Good fats

Good fats are great sources of energy and aid in nutrient absorption. Good fats include monounsaturated and polyunsaturated fats. Some of the best sources of good and healthy fats are nuts, canola, seafood, olive, soy, corn, sunflower oils, and safflower.

NOTE: Alcohol and caffeine items are not prohibited, but they are also not recommended because of their high-calorie contents. The same goes for beverages like sodas.

Below is a sample food list with more common food items:

Very Low-Energy-Dense Foods	Low-Energy-dense Foods	Medium-Energy-dense Foods	High-Energy-Dense Foods
(0-0.6 calories/gram)	(0.6-1.5 calories/gram)	(1.5-4.0 calories/gram)	(4.0-9.0 calories/gram)
Load up on: Chicken broth Broth-based soups Cucumber Celery Tomato Milk Carrots Peach Raspberries Apples	Start monitoring portion size of: Tofu Yogurt (plain, low-fat) Grapes Vegetarian chili Banana Shrimp Olives Potatoes Pasta	Control your portion size of: Frozen yogurt Eggs Turkey breast Raisins Italian dressing Bagel Hard pretzels Angel food cake Sirloin steak Ravioli	Limit your intake of: Potato chips, baked Croissant Graham crackers Granola bar Bacon Tortilla chips Peanut butter Ranch dressing Pecans

PHASE 5: PREPARING YOUR OWN FOOD WITH VOLUMETRICS DIET RECIPES

K nowing what to eat is just part of the equation of the Volumetrics Diet. You also need to learn how to prepare your food to bring out their nutrients without losing flavor.

Below are some recipes that you can follow that comply with the demands of the Volumetrics Diet. Just keep in mind that you don't have to follow these recipes to the letter. You can always change a few ingredients here and there according to your needs and budget.

Fiber One Parfait

Ingredients:
- 1/2 cup Fiber One Cereal
- 1 cup frozen mango or any fruit of your choice
- 1 cup light yogurt

Instructions:
1. Place the yogurt at the bottom of a bowl or cup and then add the fruits followed by the cereal. Repeat the steps until the bowl is full.
2. Mix the ingredients. Makes 1 serving.

Nutrition Facts:
289 Calories
4.3 grams of Total Fat
128.7 milligrams of Sodium
17.4 grams of Dietary Fiber
13.4 grams of Protein

Oatmeal Pancakes

Ingredients:
- 1-1/4 cup Quaker Oats
- 1-1/4 cup skim milk
- 1 large egg
- 1 tbsp. olive oil
- 1 cup whole wheat flour
- 1 tsp. baking powder

Instructions:
1. In a medium-size bowl, combine the cereal and the milk. Let stand for 5 minutes.
2. Add the eggs, whole wheat flour, baking powder, and olive oil. Mix well until blended.
3. Preheat a nonstick skillet, and pour 1/4 cup of the mixture. Flip and cook until it turns golden brown. Makes up to 4 servings.

Nutrition Facts per Serving:
271.3 Calories
7 grams of Total Fat
54.7 milligrams of Cholesterol
177.5 milligrams of Sodium
6.2 grams of Dietary Fiber
11.3 grams of Protein

Black Bean Soup

Ingredients:
- 2 cans black beans, drained
- 2 cups chicken broth
- 1 cup salsa

Instructions:
1. In a large pot, heat all the black beans, chicken broth, and salsa.
2. Pour the heated ingredients into a blender. Puree the black beans until creamy.
3. Garnish with herbs. Makes up to 6 servings.

Nutrition Facts per Serving:
122.7 Calories
0.6 grams of Total Fat
781.8 milligrams of Sodium
7 grams of Dietary Fiber
9.1 grams of Protein

Butternut Squash Mac and Cheese

Ingredients:
- 1 lb. Butternut squash, peeled, seeded, and diced
- 1 cup vegetable broth
- 1-1/2 cup skim milk
- nutmeg
- cayenne pepper
- 3/4 tsp. salt
- ground pepper
- 1 lb. whole wheat spirals
- 1 cup cheddar cheese, shredded
- 1/2 cup ricotta cheese
- 2 tbsp. breadcrumbs
- 1 tsp. olive oil
- olive oil cooking spray

Instructions:
1. Preheat the oven to 375 °F. Boil water in a large pot.
2. Combine squash, broth, and milk in a medium-sized saucepan. Cook the squash mixture and let it simmer for about 10 minutes.
3. Add the noodles to the boiling water. Cook the noodles for about 8 minutes.
4. Mash the squash mixture. Add nutmeg, cayenne, and season with salt and pepper. Mix well.
5. After a few minutes of cooking the noodles, drain and then mix the squash mixture. Add the cheddar, ricotta, and parmesan. Stir to combine.
6. Spray the baking dish with olive oil and then pour the noodle mixture. In a separate bowl, mix breadcrumbs, remaining parmesan, and oil. Sprinkle the mixture on top of the noodles.
7. Cover with foil. Bake for 20 minutes. After that, remove the foil and bake for another 20 minutes. Makes up to 8 servings.

Nutrition Facts per Serving:
230 Calories
4.3 grams of Total Fat

10.5 milligrams of Cholesterol
305 milligrams of Sodium
5.2 grams of Dietary Fiber
13.2 grams of Protein

Lentil Vegetable Soup

Ingredients:
- 1 cup brown lentils, dried
- 4 cups vegetable broth
- 1 can tomatoes, diced
- 2 tbsp. olive oil
- 2 garlic cloves, diced
- 1 medium onion, diced
- 2 celery stalks, chopped
- 1 bay leaf
- 2 tbsp. balsamic vinegar
- salt
- pepper

Instructions:
1. Put the lentils in a bowl, covered with water. Leave overnight.
2. In a large soup pan, cook onions using olive oil over medium heat. Add garlic and celery. Once the celery begins to soften, add tomatoes, carrots, and vegetable broth. Add the lentils.
3. Bring the mixture to a boil then put the heat to medium-low. Let it simmer for 30 minutes.
4. Discard bay leaf and then add vinegar. Season with salt and pepper to taste. Makes 4 servings.

Nutrition Facts per Serving:
228. 7 Calories
9.1 grams of Total Fat
1082 milligrams of Sodium
6.7 grams of Dietary Fiber
7.9 grams of Protein

Rustic Tomato Lentil Soup

Ingredients:
- 1 medium-sized onion, diced
- 3 medium carrots, chopped
- 2 tbsp. olive oil
- 2 celery stalks , minced
- 6 cups vegetable broth
- 1 can tomatoes, diced
- 2 cups cooked lentils
- 1 cup dry pasta
- pepper
- cayenne pepper

Instructions:
1. Sauté garlic, onions, and carrots in a large soup pot. Use medium-high heat. When the onions are translucent, add vegetable broth, celery, lentils, pepper, and cayenne, and bring to a boil.
2. Reduce the heat to medium-low and let the soup simmer for around 10 minutes. Add the pasta and cook for another 10 minutes. Makes 4 servings.

Nutrition Facts per Serving:
243.9 Calories
8 grams of Total Fat
235.8 milligrams of Sodium
8.8 grams of Dietary Fiber
8.8 grams of Protein

Chicken Citrus Salad

Ingredients:
- 2 tbsp. orange juice, fresh
- 2 tbsp. red wine vinegar
- 2 tsp. Olive oil
- 2 tsp. honey
- 1 ¼ tsp. Dijon-style mustard
- 4 small skinless, boneless chicken breasts, halves
- 4 cups mixed salad greens
- 2 medium oranges, peeled and sectioned
- 8 strawberries

Instructions:
1. Combine orange juice, red wine vinegar, olive oil, honey, and mustard in a medium-sized mixing bowl. Set aside.
2. Grill chicken for 6 minutes over medium-hot coals. Turn the chicken and grill until tender.
3. Combine the mixed greens and orange in a large bowl. Toss to mix.
4. Arrange the salad on a plate. Place chicken on the side. Drizzle with the vinaigrette. Garnish with strawberries. Makes 4 servings.

Nutrition Facts per Serving:
211.4 Calories
3.9 grams of Total Fat
49.3 milligrams of Cholesterol
84.1 milligrams of Sodium
5.4 grams of Dietary Fiber
22.1 grams of Protein

Red White and Blue Trifle

Ingredients:
- 1 carton low-fat Ricotta cheese (15-oz)
- 1 carton fat-free lemon (6-oz)
- 1/2 cup powdered sugar
- 2 tsp. vanilla extract
- 1 round angel food cake (10 inch), cut into 1-inch cubes
- 1 medium banana
- 2 tsp. lemon juice
- 2 cups unsweetened wild blueberries, frozen
- 2 cups fresh blackberries
- 2 cups fresh strawberries, sliced
- 1-1/2 cups fat-free whipped topping, frozen

Instructions:
1. Place the ricotta, yogurt, sugar, and vanilla in a blender. Blend until smooth. Set aside.
2. Layer one-third of the cake cubes in the bottom of a deep bowl. Pour one-third of the ricotta mixture evenly over the cubes.
3. Combine the peeled and sliced banana with the orange juice by tossing. Layer one-third of it over the ricotta mixture. Repeat the process.
4. Spread the whipped topping over the fruit layer. Cover and refrigerate for 2 hours. Makes 15 servings.

Nutrition Facts per Serving:
152.5 Calories
1.3 grams of Total Fat
7.3 milligrams of Cholesterol
50.3 milligrams of Sodium
3.2 grams of Dietary Fiber
5 grams of Protein

White Bean Tapenade

Ingredients:
- 2 garlic cloves, unpeeled
- 1/2 tsp. olive oil
- 1 15-oz.can Cannellini beans, drained and rinsed
- 2 tsp. lemon juice
- 2 tbsp. Olive oil
- 6 sage leaves, fresh
- salt
- pepper

Instructions:
1. Preheat the oven to 350°F. Wrap the garlic cloves in foil after drizzling them with olive oil. Place the wrapped garlic in the oven until soft, about 30 minutes.
2. Let it cool down and then remove the skin from the garlic.
3. Combine all the ingredients except the sage leaves in a blender; process until soft.
4. Chop the sage leaves thinly and then fold them into a tapenade. Add more seasonings if desired. Makes up to 12 servings.

Nutrition Facts per Serving:
50 Calories
2.6 grams of Total Fat
0 milligrams of Cholesterol
54.9 milligrams of Sodium
1.6 grams of Dietary Fiber
2 grams of Protein

Turkey Chili with Corn and Black Beans

Ingredients:
- 20 oz. Ground Turkey
- 1 medium-sized onion, minced
- 1 medium-sized red bell pepper, chopped
- 2 tbsp. chili powder
- 1 tbsp. cumin
- 1 tsp. oregano
- 1 tbsp. red pepper flakes
- 1 can tomatoes with juice, diced
- 1 small can tomato sauce
- 1 can yellow corn
- 1 can black beans, rinsed
- 1 can seasoned chili beans

Instructions:
1. Place the ground turkey in a hot large skillet or pot. After a few minutes, add the minced onions, red bell pepper, chili powder, cumin, oregano, and red pepper flakes.
2. Cook the turkey until tender and no longer pinkish. After that, add the tomato sauce and juice, yellow corn, black beans, and chili beans.
3. Reduce heat to medium-low and then cover the pot. Let it simmer for 30 to 45 minutes or until other ingredients are cooked.
4. Add any toppings of your choice. Makes up to 8 servings.

Nutrition Facts per Serving:
212.6 Calories
6.4 grams of Total Fat
0 milligrams of Cholesterol
361.5 milligrams of Sodium
6.1 grams of Dietary Fiber
19.4 grams of Protein

Eggs-n-Oats

Ingredients:
- 1 large egg
- 2 egg whites
- 1/2 cup Quaker oats
- 2 oz. skim milk

Instructions:
1. Combine all the ingredients in a medium-sized mixing bowl. Combine well.
2. Preheat a nonstick pan and spray with cooking oil.
3. Pour the mixture into the pan. Scramble as you would with ordinary eggs.
4. Add more seasonings if you like. You can top it with banana, honey, berries, or cinnamon. 1 serving only.

Nutrition Facts per Serving:
272.6 Calories
8 grams of Total Fat
187 milligrams of Cholesterol
201.6 milligrams of Sodium
4 grams of Dietary Fiber
20.2 grams of Protein

Southwest Pasta Salad

Ingredients:
- 1 box whole-wheat pasta, 8-ounce
- 1 can corn, 15-ounce
- 1 can black beans, 15-ounce
- 1 cup salsa
- 1 cup low-fat cheddar cheese, shredded
- 1 cup green bell pepper, diced
- garlic powder
- cayenne pepper
- 1 cup tomatoes, chopped

Instructions:
1. Cook pasta according to package instructions. After cooking, drain, rinse, and place in a large bowl. Set aside.
2. Drain and reserve the liquids from the canned corn and black beans.
3. Combine the salsa, cheese, green pepper, tomatoes, canned corn, and black beans in the pasta. Mix well. Add a small amount of the liquid from the canned corn and beans.
4. Cover and refrigerate. Makes up to 8 servings.

Nutrition Facts per Serving:
267.8 Calories
3.3 grams of Total Fat
3 milligrams of Cholesterol
546.5 milligrams of Sodium
7 grams of Dietary Fiber
14.2 grams of Protein

Cabbage Vegetable Soup

Ingredients:
- 1 can crushed tomatoes, 28-oz
- 1 onion, diced
- 3 celery stalks , diced
- 3 medium carrots, diced
- 1 head cabbage, shredded
- 1 can green beans, 14.5-oz
- 1 can sweet yellow corn, 12-oz
- 1 can pinto beans, 15-oz

Instructions:
1. Place the tomatoes, onion, celery, carrots, and cabbage in a large pot.
2. Cook for a few minutes and then let it simmer over medium-low heat until the vegetables are soft. This will take around 20 minutes.
3. Add the green beans, yellow corn, and pinto beans.
4. Let it simmer for another 5 minutes. Add salt and pepper to taste. Makes up to 6 servings.

Nutrition Facts per Serving:
165.2 Calories
1.8 grams of Total Fat
0 milligrams of Cholesterol
273.5 milligrams of Sodium
12 grams of Dietary Fiber
8.3 grams of Protein

PHASE 6: PREPARING A VOLUMETRICS MEAL PLAN

The Volumetrics diet plan does not prohibit any type of food, but it recommends moderation of certain categories of food such as the medium-density and high-density foods. The plan focuses on the science of satiety and behavior modification. To stay satiated, energy-density foods were introduced. Energy density is the number of calories a food has per volume. With this, food with high water content is recommended.

The diet plan does not only focus on the management of calories; it also recommends foods with other nutrients. Protein is one important nutrient because it takes more time to digest and it makes you feel fuller for a longer time. Other nutrients such as complex carbohydrates and fiber are also very important.

A meal plan must span the entire day which means that it should include breakfast, lunch, and dinner. Snacks are also to be included but must appear in the plan once per day. With that in mind, here is an example of a Volumetrics Meal Plan.

Breakfast

Oatmeal topped with banana, cinnamon, and brown sugar.
Non-fat milk
1 cup honeydew melon

Lunch
Autumn Harvest pumpkin soup
Whole wheat pita bread
1/2 cup sugar-free chocolate pudding
Strawberries

Dinner
Steak fajita with grilled green peppers and onions, salsa, diced fresh tomato, and corn kernels
"Minted" broccoli

Snacks
8 oz. low-fat blueberry yogurt
Cheerios with skim milk and strawberries

To reach your goals using the Volumetrics eating plan, you have to always find a way to minimize your meal's energy density. Adding more water-rich and fiber-rich ingredients is one way of reducing energy density. Eating lean protein promotes fullness, which means that your food intake will also decrease. Another strategy to maintain fullness is to add fruits and vegetables to every meal. Instead of eating Cheerios, eat more watery fruits.

The key point of an effective Volumetrics meal plan is to divide the required daily calorie consumption per meal. You must first calculate your required daily calorie intake and reduce it by 500 to 1000 calories depending on your weight loss goal. The usual calorie intake ranges from 1600 to 2400 calories per day.

CONCLUSION

After all, is said and done, the biggest question you might have is this:

Is the Volumetrics plan really effective?

The answer is a resounding YES. If you look at the Volumetrics diet plan in the most basic of terms possible, it simply requires you to be sensible with the food that you eat. This means that you have to cut down on unnecessary calories as well as unhealthy forms of fat.

I recommend checking out Barbara Rolls' full list of books on this diet plan for a much more detailed overview of this diet plan.

It is not as bombastic as other weight loss plans since it does not promise massive losses in a short period of time. Instead, what it does assure is that you will learn how to pick your food more carefully over a period of time. This will eventually help you improve your body as it burns through all that stored fat efficiently.

This plan is ideal for anyone who wants to eat healthier and would like to prepare their own food. With a few recipes that are in line with your weight loss goals, this diet plan should help you gradually shed off all that unnecessary fat and achieve a better physique.

REFERENCES AND HELPFUL LINKS

Insight, F. (2019, June 26). The basics of the volumetrics diet. Food Insight. https://foodinsight.org/basics-of-volumetrics-diet/.

Volumetrics diet review: Does it work for weight loss? (2020, August 11). Healthline. https://www.healthline.com/nutrition/volumetrics-diet.

What is the volumetrics diet? (n.d.). Verywell Fit. Retrieved May 6, 2023, from https://www.verywellfit.com/the-volumetrics-diet-what-you-need-to-know-3496210.

What is the volumetrics diet? (2022, October 13). Cleveland Clinic. https://health.clevelandclinic.org/volumetrics-diet/.

Zelman, K. M., RD, LD, MPH, & Schweitzer, L. (n.d.). Volumetrics diet plan review: Foods and effectiveness. WebMD. Retrieved May 6, 2023, from https://www.webmd.com/diet/a-z/volumetrics-what-it-is.